NMADA receptors and anesthesia

Author :Hala Mostafa Goma .MD.

Professor of Anesthesia ,Faculty of medicine,Cairo University.

Ahmeda1995@yahoo.com

TABLE OF CONTENT

Introduction:

WHAT IS NMDA RECEPTORS

- NMDAR is a specific type of ionotropic glutamate receptor.

- Agonist molecule N-methyl-D-aspartate (NMDA) binds selectively to the NMDA receptor.

- **Mechanism of action of NMADA receptors**

  NMDA receptor is voltage-dependent activation, with a reversal potential near 0 mV. Stimulation of NMDA receptors results in the opening of nonselective ion gates to cations. That leads to blocking of the ion channels by extracellular Mg^{2+} & Zn^{2+} ions. This leads to the flow of Na^+, and small amounts of Ca^{2+} ions into the cell and K^+.

  Synaptic plasticity: defined as Calcium flux through NMDARs .which is essential for learning and memory.

  The NMDA receptor is stimulated by two methods:

  1-It is ligand-gated and voltage-dependent.

  Second:

  2- It requires co-activation by two ligands: glutamate and either D-serine or glycine.

  Pharamacological NMADA agonist:

- psychoactive drugs such as phencyclidine (PCP),

- Alcohol (ethanol) and dextromethorphan(DXM).

- The anesthetic drugs ketamine and nitrous oxide are partially because of their effects on NMDA receptor activity.

STRUCURE OF NMADA RECEPTORS:

- The NMDA receptor combination heterotetramer between two GluN1 and two GluN2 subunits (NR1 and NR2),

- Two essential NR1 subunits and two regionally localized NR2 subunits.

- A related gene family of NR3 A and B subunits has an inhibitory effect on receptor activity.

- Multiple receptor isoforms have brain distributions, and functional properties arise by difference between the NR1 transcripts, and the NR2 subunits.

- Each receptor subunit has special design, and each structural

- design as well represents a functional unit:

- The *extracellular domain* contains two major structures:

- a modulatory domain and a ligand-binding domain.

- NR1 subunits bind the co-agonist glycine and NR2 subunits bind the neurotransmitter glutamate.

- The agonist-binding module binds to a membrane domain, which consists of three trans-membrane segments ,and a re-entrant loop reminiscent of the selectivity filter of potassium channels.

- **The membrane domain contributes to the channel pore ,and is responsible for** :

- High-unitary conductance,

- High-calcium permeability,

- Voltage -dependent magnesium block.

- Each subunit has an extensive cytoplasmic domain, which contain residues that can be directly modified by a series of protein kinases ,and protein phosphatases, as well as interact with a large number of structural, adaptor, and scaffolding proteins.

- The glycine-binding modules of the NR1 and NR3 subunits, and the glutamate-binding module of the NR2A subunit are soluble proteins, and they are three-dimensional structure, and solved at atomic resolution by x-ray crystallography.

- This forms a common fold with amino acid-binding bacterial proteins with the glutamate-binding module of AMPA-receptors, and kainate-receptors.

Dynamic property of NMADA recptors:

- The NMDA receptors are a non-selective channesl that can allow the passage of Ca^{2+} and Na^+ into the cell and K^+ out of the cell.

- The excitatory postsynaptic potential (EPSP) produced by activation of an NMDA receptor increases the concentration of Ca^{2+} (second messenger) in the cell.

- However, the NMDA receptor cation channel is blocked by Mg^{2+} at resting membrane potential. Depolariza tion unblock the channel.

Coincidence detector:

The NMDA receptor functions as a "molecular . Its ion channel opens only when

- Glutamate is bound to the receptor, and the postsynaptic cell is depolarized (which removes the Mg^{2+} blocking the channel).

NMDA receptors are modulation:

- endogenous,
  1- Na^+, K^+ and Ca^{2+} not only pass through the NMDA receptor channel but also modulate the activity of NMDA receptors.
  2- Zn^{2+} and Cu^{2+} generally block NMDA current activity in a noncompetitive and a voltage-independent .

3- Pb^{2+} is a potent NMDAR antagonist. Presynaptic deficits resulting from Pb^{2+} exposure during synaptogenesis are mediated by disruption of NMDAR-dependent BDNF signaling.

4- Kynurenic acid is an endogenous NMDA receptor antagonist.

5- H^+ concentration control the activity of NMDA receptors is also strongly sensitive to the changes in, and incompletely inhibited by the ambient concentration of H^+ under physiological conditions.

6- Redox modulatory site NMDA receptor function is also strongly regulated by chemical reduction and oxidation, reductants severely enhance NMDA channel activity, whereas oxidants either reverse the effects of reductants or depress native responses. It is generally believed that NMDA receptors are modulated by endogenous redox agents such as glutathione, lipoic acid, and the essential nutrient pyrroloquinoline quinone.

7- Src kinase enhances NMDA receptor currents.

8- Reelin modulates NMDA function through Src family kinases and DAB1.

9- CDK5 regulates the amount of NR2B-containing NMDA receptors on the synaptic membrane.

NMDA Receptors Agonists:

- Activation of NMDA receptors requires binding of glutamate or aspartate.

- NMDARs also require the binding of the co-agonist <u>glycine</u> for the efficient opening of the ion channel.

- D-serine has also been found to co-agonize the NMDA receptor with even greater potency than glycine.

- D-serine is produced by serine racemase, and is enriched in the same areas as NMDA receptors.

- Removal of D-serine can block NMDA-mediated excitatory neurotransmission in many areas.

- Recently, it has been shown that D-serine can be released both by neurons, and astrocytes to regulate NMDA receptors.

NMDA receptor agonists include:

- Aminocyclopropanecarboxylic acid.
- D-Cycloserine.
- cis-2,3-Piperidinedicarboxylic acid.
- Aspartic acid.
- Glutamic acid.
- Quinolinate.
- Homocysteic acid.

- D-Serine.
- L-Serine.
- D-Alanine.
- L-Alanine.
- ACPL

Partial agonists.

- N-Methyl-D-aspartic acid (NMDA)
- 3,5-dibromo-L-phenylalanine[22]
- **Rapastinel (GLYX-13)**
  - Rapastinel, and NRX-1074Glycine-site NMDA receptor partial agonists are now studied with great interest for the development of new drugs with antidepressant and analgesic effects without obvious psychotomimetic activities.

NMADA Antagonists:

Antagonists of the NMDA receptor are used as

- anesthetics for animals and sometimes humans,
- recreational drugs due to their hallucinogenic properties,
- dissociation
- Olney's lesions. brain damage : When certain NMDA receptor antagonists are given to rodents in large doses asm ketamine, phencyclidine, and dextrorphan (a metabolite of dextromethorphan

NMDA receptor antagonists used in research environments.

- AP5
- Conantokins
- Dextromethorphan
- Dexanabinol
- Dizocilpine (MK-801)
- Ketamine
- Memantine
- Nitrous oxide
- Phencyclidine
- Xenon

Weak NMDA receptor antagonism is a secondary or additional action include:

- Amantadine
- Atomoxetine
- Dextropropoxyphene
- Ethanol
- Huperzine A
- Ibogaine
- Ketobemidone
- Methadone – an opioid analgesic
- Tramadol – an atypical analgesic

- It has been demonstrated that polyamines do not directly activate NMDA receptors, but instead act to potentiate or inhibit glutamate-mediated responses.

- Amino glycosides have neurotoxic drug.

The role of the NMDA receptor in memory, and learning

NMDA receptor (NMDAR)-mediated currents are directly related to membrane depolarization. NMDA agonists therefore exhibit fast Mg^{2+} unbinding kinetics, increasing channel open probability with depolarization, this channel is a biochemical substrate of Hebbian learning, where it can act as a coincidence detector for membrane depolarization and synaptic transmission.

Anesthesia, and NMDA Receptors

1-preoperative preparation and special concern for patients receiving NMADA antagonists as

- Alzheimer patients. Memantine is an NMDA receptor antagonist used in the treatment of Alzheimer's disease
- Psychosis patients.
- Parkinsonism.
- Aminoglycosides.

Neurotoxicty after pronged use of NMADA antagonists:

NMDA receptor antagonists aretherapeutic agents for the treatment of neurological disorders such as stroke, epilepsy, pain and Parkinson's disease.

These compounds cause adverse behavioral (psychotomimetic) effects ,and can produce neurotoxicity characterized

1 neuronal vacuolization,
2 induction of heat-shock protein,
3 neuronal/axonal degeneration
4 Regional brain cell death in several animal species.

NMDA antagonists induce neurotoxicity in humans.

- The mechanism of NMDA antagonist-induced neurotoxicity is not completely known.
- Evidence suggests disinhibition of GABAergic inputs to the affected neurons.

- Several classes of compounds have been shown to prevent NMDA antagonist-induced neurotoxicity. T

Factors affecting the extent of neurotoxicity produced by NMDA antagonists are:

Type of antagonist

Dose,

Exposure length.

Anesthetic consideration of NMADA receptors antagonists:

1- Local anesthetics, bupivacine, ropivacaine.

2- Ketamine, s ketamine.

3- Magnesium.

4- Tramadol with special concern with tramadol addiction.

5- Nitrous oxide anesthesia.

6- Xenon anesthesia.

7- Synergetic effect between local anesthetics and s ketamine leads to decrease dose of local anesthetics.

8- Increase analgesia in regional block, brachial nerve blockade ,and phantom limbs .

9- Decrease dose of narcotics as morphine in prolonged infusion in cancer patients.

10- Potentiating by using combination of NMADA receptors decreases risk of addiction.

11-   Dextromethorphan, a synthetic analogue of codeine, the d-isomer of 3-methoxy-N-methylmorphine

Role of the NMDA receptor in anesthesia:

cascade of sensitization dorsal horn:

- NMDA receptor activation triggers of events leading to dynamic neurones.
- There is a significant increase in intracellular calcium and activation of protein kinases and phosphorylating enzymes.
- NMDA receptor stimulation will also increase the production of spinal phospholipase ,and induce the production of nitric oxide synthetase.
- The prostaglandins and nitric oxide which are subsequently produced and released into the extracellular milieu can facilitate further release of excitatory amino acids and neuropeptides from primary afferent pain fibres.
- The NMDA receptor antagonists ketamine and dextromethorphan can block this cascade of events which contribute to sensitisation.
- NMDA receptors mediate excitatory neurotransmission in brain and spinal cord and play a critical role in the neurological disease state of chronic pain, which is caused by central sensitization.

Local anesthetics ,and NMADAR antagonism:

- Most local anesthetic agents consist of a lipophilic group (aromatic benzene ring) connected by an intermediate chain via an ester or amide linkage to an ionizable group (e.g., a tertiary amine). Local anesthetics may therefore be classified as aminoester or aminoamide compounds.

- The amino-ester local anesthetics are: procaine, chlorprocaine and tetracaine. The amino-amides consist of lidocaine, mepivacaine, prilocaine, bupivacaine, and etidocaine.

- The ester and amide local anesthetics differ in their chemical stability, biotransformation, and allergic potential. Amides are extremely stable agents, while esters are relatively unstable in solution.

- Local anesthetics are weak bases ,and are made available clinically as salts to increase their solubility and stability. Inside the body they exist as the uncharged base (unionized form) or as a cation (ionized form). The relative proportions of these two forms are governed by the pKa specific for each local anesthetic and the pH of the body fluids.   .

Mechanism of Action of Bupivicaine:

- The primary mechanism of action of bupivacaine is blockage of voltage-gated sodium channels. The excitable membrane of nerve axons like the membrane of cardiac muscle fibres and neuronal cell bodies maintains a resting membrane potential of -90 to -60 mV. During excitation the sodium channels open and fast inward sodium current quickly depolarizes the membrane towards the sodium equilibrium potential (+40 mV).

- As a result of depolarization, the sodium channels close (inactivate) and potassium channels open. The outward flow of potassium repolarizes the membrane towards the potassium equilibrium potential (about -90 mV) repolarization returns the membrane to the resting state. The trans-membrane ionic gradients are maintained by the sodium pump.

- Thus, there appears to be a single binding site for local anesthetics on the sodium channel. Sodium currents are reduced by local anesthetics because the drug-bound channels fail to open. Inactivation and anesthetic binding prevent the conformational changes that constitute the activation process by fully or partially immobilizing the channel. Pain impulses fail to traverse the drugged axon. Impulse activity entering the anesthetized region thus maintains its own failure.

- Bupivacaine is the indicated local anesthetic in caudal, epidural, and spinal anesthesia and is widely used clinically to manage acute and chronic pain.

- In addition to blocking Na^+ channels, bupivacaine affects the activity of many other channels, including NMDA receptors. Importantly, bupivacaine inhibits NMDA receptor-mediated synaptic transmission in the dorsal horn of the spinal cord, an area critically involved in central sensitization.

- There is inhibition state-independent inhibition because it occurred to the same degree whether the drug was mediated by extracellular and intracellular inhibitory sites, via hydrophilic and hydrophobic pathways.

- These results predict that clinical doses of bupivacaine would decrease the peak, and accelerate the decay of synaptic NMDA receptor currents during normal synaptic transmission.

- These quantitative predictions inform possible applications of bupivacaine as preventative and therapeutic approaches in chronic pain.

Magnesium sulphate ,and NMADAR antagonism:

- Intravenous magnesium sulphate alters pain processing and reduces the induction and maintenance of central sensitization by non-competitively through its action on Ethyl-D-aspartate (NMDA) receptors in the spinal cord, and this can be explained by analgesic, and anti inflammatory effects.

- NMDA antagonists reduce the excitability of nociceptive input terminals of C-fibres that play a role in the central processing of pain.

- Magnesium has been shown to reduce post-operative analgesic requirements

- Intra-operative intravenous magnesium sulphate at very high doses has been reported to reduce postoperative morphine consumption, but not post-operative pain scores.

- It was reported that intravenous magnesium (3.0 – 3.5 g) can be a useful adjuvant in intraoperative analgesia,

- The exact dose needs to be determined. Since the magnesium ion poorly crosses the blood—brain barrier in humans,

- Antagonist properties of magnesium ion in the CNS,

- intrathecal magnesium sulphate has been shown to potentiate morphine antinociception in a postoperative pain model.

- It has also been shown that co-administration of magnesium sulphate with ropivacaine for post-operative infiltration analgesia after radical retropubic prostatectomy produces a significant reduction in tramadole requirements

- Magnesium sulphate combined with bupivacaine produced a reduction in postoperative pain, when given intra-articularly, in comparison with either bupivacaine or magnesium alone, or with saline placebo.

- Magnesium sulphate can provide analgesia when administered intra-articularly for arthroscopic surgery.

- In addition, NMDA receptors are present in the peripheral terminal of articular primary afferent fibres in the knee joint and on cellular elements within the joint, such as synoviocytes and immune cells,

- and their activation has been found potentially to play a role in nociception.

- Considering this evidence, many authors were interested to investigate whether magnesium sulphate had beneficial effects in TKA, one of the most painful surgical procedures in orthopaedics.

- The analgesic effect of intra-articular magnesium sulphate and ropivacaine mixture was evident. They cocluded that a local effect was at least partially responsible for this as the side-effects usually seen after systemic administration of magnesium sulphate were not observed.

- Low concentrations of intra-articular magnesium and ropivacaine provided efficient pain relief In conclusion, an intra-operative intra-articular injection of magnesium sulphate and ropivacaine during TKA can reduce the post-operative morphine analgesic requirements with no adverse events. These results demonstrate that a magnesium sulphate and ropivacaine mixture could be used as an adjuvant therapy for postoperative analgesic management.

TRMADOL

- **Tramadol** (marketed as **Ultram**,) is an opioid pain medication which is used to treat moderate to moderately severe pain.

- When taken as an immediate-release oral formulation, the onset of pain relief usually occurs within about an hour.

Mechanisms of action of trmadol.

- First, it binds to the μ-opioid receptor.

- Second, it inhibits the reuptake of serotonin, and nor epinephrine.

Side effects of tramadol:

1- seizures, increased risk of serotonin syndrome,

2- Decreased alertness.

3- Drug addiction.

4- Common side effects include: constipation, itchiness and nausea, among others.

5- A change in dosage may be recommended in those with kidney or liver problems. Its use is not recommended in women who are breast feeding or those who are at risk of suicide.

Serotonin syndrome

- Serotonin sickness, serotonin storm, serotonin poisoning, hyperserotonemia, or serotonergic syndrome.

- It is a potential symptom combination, overdose of tramadol, or the Serotonin syndrome is not an idiopathic drug reaction; it is a predictable consequence of excess serotonin on the CNS and/or peripheral nervous system. For this reason, some experts strongly prefer the terms **serotonin toxicity** or **serotonin toxidrome**

- Symptoms including cognitive, autonomic, and somatic effects. Symptoms may range from barely perceptible to fatal

- gitated delirium; dry oral mucosa; hot, dry, erythematous skin; urinary retention; and an absence of bowel sounds. Hyperactive bowel sounds — along with neuromuscular abnormalities, diaphoresis, and normal skin color.

- Differential diagnosis ,malignant hyper thermia ,over dose of anticholinergics.

- Diagnosis includes observing symptoms and investigating patient history for causal factors (interacting drugs).

- No laboratory tests can currently confirm the diagnosis

- Hence it is diagnosed based on symptoms, disease course (that is, the progression of the disease) and the exclusion of other possible causes of the presenting symptoms.

Treatment of serotonin syndrome:

- Treatment consists of discontinuing medications which may contribute and in moderate to severe cases administering a

  ### Serotonin antagonists.

  - Cyproheptadine blocks 5-HT$_{2A}$, HI and is a mild anticholinergic.

  - Methysergide is a 5-HT$_{2A}$ antagonist and nonselective 5-HT$_1$ receptor blocker. It causes retroperitoneal fibrosis and mediastinal fibrosis.

  - Quetiapine blocks 5-HT$_{2A}$, 5-HT$_{1A}$, dopamine receptors D$_1$ and D$_2$, histamine receptor H1, and A1 adrenoreceptors.

  - An important adjunct treatment includes controlling agitation with benzodiazepine sedation.

Clinical use of tramadol

1. Tramadol is marketed as a racemic mixture of both *R*- and *S*-stereoisomers. This is because the two isomers complement each other's analgesic activity. It is often combined with paracetamol as this is known to improve the efficacy of tramadol in relieving pain.

2. Itraoperative itravenously,post operatively IV,IM,orally.

3. Regionally in spinal, epidural anesthesia, and with lidocaine intravenous regional anesthesia.

Metabolism of tramadol

- Tramadol is metabolised to *O*-desmethyltramadol, which is a more potent opioid . It is of the benzenoid class.

Tramadol/Ultram Addiction

- Tramadol/Ultram is an atypical opiate which is a centrally acting analgesic used for treating moderate to severe pain.

- It is a synthetic agent.

- Tramadol is available in injectable, intravenous and/or intramuscular and oral preparations. When combined with acetaminophen, it is identified as Ultracet.

Unlike most other opioids,

- Tramadol/ULTRAM is not considered a controlled substance in many countries (the U.S. and Australia, among others) and is available with a normal prescription. Tramadol is also available over-the-counter without prescription in a few countries.

- Tramadol is sometimes mistakenly classified as a non-opioid analgesic, because its abuse liability is lower than that of other opioids and because it has multiple mechanisms of action (not only, but including, mu-opioid activity).

- Tramadol is used to treat moderate and severe pain and most types of neuralgia.

- Ultram/Tramadol is often prescribed by physicians that do not realize that this drug is very addicting. It usually alleviates pain, at least to a tolerable level, and it feels safe to take this medication as needed without the worry of dependence.

- This is where the insidious nature of Ultram is revealed. It turns out, that despite the initial belief that this medication does not pose the risk of dependency, this is unfortunately not the case.

- Ultram has proven to be one of the most habit-forming and addictive medications on the market. As is the case with opiate drugs, when use is discontinued abruptly, the body reacts by withdrawing in a violent and sometimes dangerous manner.

- For those who treat their physical and emotional discomfort with Ultram, withdrawal from this drug is one of the most horrible and unbearable to experience comparable to that of withdrawal from heroin.

- This is an added factor in continuing use of the drug resulting in the aforementioned drug-seeking behavior usually seen with the opiate medications.

- The maximum allowed dosage during a 24-hour time period is 400 milligrams which equates to eight 50mg tablets. Patients are known to abuse Ultram to the extent that they ingest 20 to 30 and more of the 50mg tablets per day.

- Many doctors are still not aware of this danger and continue to prescribe without warning to patients of its extreme habit-forming potential. Though some doctors and practices have learned about this through patient experiences and have begun to treat Ultram with the same care and restrictiveness as other opiate pain medications.

- Tramadol/Ultram is marketed as an analgesic medication with a weak affinity for the opioid receptor (approximately 1/6th that of morphine)

Tramadol/Ultram Addiction Effects

Adverse drug reactions are:

- Nausea,

- Vomiting

- Sweating.

- Drowsiness, it is less of an issue than for other opioids.

- Respiratory depression, a common side effect of most opioids, is not clinically significant in normal doses.

- By itself, it can decrease the seizure threshold. Dosages of coumadin/warfarin may need to be reduced for anticoagulated patients to avoid bleeding complications.

- Some controversy exists regarding the dependence liability of tramadol. Grünenthal has promoted it as an opioid with a lower risk of opioid dependence than that of traditional opioids claiming little evidence of such dependence in clinical trials.

- Despite these claims, it is apparent in community practice that dependence to this agent does occur. Nevertheless, the prescribed information for Ultram warns that tramadol "may induce psychological and physical dependence of the morphine-type". In addition, there are widespread reports by consumers of extremely difficult withdrawal experiences.

Anesthesia and tramadol addiction:

1-Determine stage of tramadol use:

- **Tolarence**

- **Physical dependence.**

- **addiction**

2-preoperative evaluation:

Organ damage, infectious diseases such as human immunodeficiency virus, tuberculosis, hepatitis, associated psychological disorders.

3- Postoperative pain management:

Tolerance

Tolerance, as defined by either of the following:

1. A need for markedly increased amounts of the substance to get the desired effect

2. Markedly diminished effect with continued use of the same amount of the substance.

3. Withdrawal symptoms,

   The same (or a closely related) substance is taken to relieve or avoid withdrawal symptoms.

   4. The substance is often taken in larger amounts or over a longer period than was planned

   5. There is a persistent desire or unsuccessful efforts to reduce or control substance use .

   6. more time is spent in activities preoperative necessary to get the substance, use the substance, or recover from its effects

   7. social, occupational, or recreational activities are reduced because of substance use.

   8. The substance use is continued despite knowledge of having a persistent or recurrent physical or psychological problem .

Physiologic dependence:

no evidence of tolerance or withdrawal

Criteria for opioid withdrawal

1- Cessation of (or reduction in) opioid use that has been heavy and prolonged (several weeks or longer)

2- Administration of an opioid antagonist after a period of opioid use B. Three (or more) 3- Dysphoric mood

 4- Nausea or vomiting

5-Muscle aches

6- Lacrimation or rhinorrhea

7- Pupillary dilation,

8- piloerection, or

9- sweating

10- Diarrhea

11- Yawning

12- Fever

13- Insomnia

pre operative pain management:

1-consultation of addiction specialists for perioperative planning

2-history for previous surgery, trauma, the need for more opiod , in suffiency of postoperative analgesia.

3- Reassurance to relieve anxiety and the fear against pain ,anxiolytics may be needed.

Intraoperative anesthestic consideration.

Maintain baseline opioids

Increase intraoperative

Provide peripheral neural or plexus blockade

nonopioids as analgesic adjuncts, as s ketamine.

Post operative consideration:

1-Put aplan or stragey for post operative pain control:

2-postoperative opioid dose to compensate for tolerance(oral, transdermal, intravenous)

3-consider neuraxial analgesic techniques when clinically indicated.

4-Maintain baseline opioids.

5 Use multiple analgesic techniques.

6. Patient-controlled analgesia: Use as primary therapy or as supplementation for epidural or regional techniques.

5. Continue neuraxial opioids: intrathecal or epidural analgesia.

6. Continue continuous neural blockade. After discharge

7. If surgery provides complete pain relief, opioids should be slowly decreased than suddenly discontinued.

8-Arrange for a timely outpatient pain clinic follow-up or a visit with the patient's addictionologist.

S KETAMINE

S ketamine is NMADAR antagonist , it also blocks dopamine receptors.

- Sketamine is approximately twice as potent as <u>racemic</u> ketamine.

- It is eliminated from the human body more quickly than R(−)-ketamine or racemic ketamine, although R(−)-ketamine slows its elimination.

- A number of studies have suggested that S ketamine has a more medically useful pharmacological action than R(−)-ketamine or racemic ketamine.

- S ketamine inhibits dopamine transporters eight times more than R(−)-ketamine.

- This increases dopamine activity in the brain. At doses causing the same intensity of effects.

- S ketamine is generally considered to be more pleasant by patients. Patients also generally recover mental function more quickly after being treated with pure S ketamine, which may be a result of the fact that it is cleared from their system more quickly.

- S ketamine has an affinity for the PCP binding site of the NMDA receptor 3-4 times higher than that of R (−)-ketamine. Unlike R(−)-ketamine,

- ketamine does not bind significantly to <u>sigma receptors</u>.

- S ketamine increases glucose metabolism in <u>frontal cortex</u>, while R(−)-ketamine decreases glucose metabolism in the brain. This difference may be responsible for the fact that esketamine generally has a more dissociative or <u>hallucinogenic</u> effect while R (−)-ketamine is reportedly more relaxing.

- However, other studies have found no difference between the isomers in the patient's level of vigilance.

- S-ketamine as an anesthetic adjuvant to propofol on treatment response to electroconvulsive therapy in treatment-resistant depression

- S ketamine is used of sub-anesthetic intravenous and adjuvant dexmedetomidine when treating acute pain from CRPS.

- Intravenous S ketamine infusion is as an adjuvant to morphine severe cancer pain from metastatic neuroblastoma.

Refernces:

1. Laube B, Hirai H, Sturgess M, Betz H, Kuhse J (1997). "Molecular determinants of agonist discrimination by NMDA receptor subunits: analysis of the glutamate binding site on the NR2B subunit". *Neuron* **18** (3): 493–503.

2. Li F, Tsien JZ (2009). "Memory and the NMDA receptors". *N. Engl. J. Med.* **361** (3): 302–3

3. Dingledine R, Borges K, Bowie D, Traynelis SF (March 1999). "The glutamate receptor ion channels". *Pharmacol. Rev.* **51** (1): 7–61.

4. Liu Y, Zhang J (October 2000). "Recent development in NMDA receptors". *Chin. Med. J.* **113** (10): 948–56.

5. Cull-Candy S, Brickley S, Farrant M (June 2001). "NMDA receptor subunits: diversity, development and disease". *Curr. Opin. Neurobiol.* **11** (3): 327–35.

6. Paoletti P, Neyton J (February 2007). "NMDA receptor subunits: function and pharmacology". *Curr Opin Pharmacol* **7** (1): 39–

7. Kleckner NW, Dingledine R (August 1988). "Requirement for glycine in activation of NMDA-receptors expressed in Xenopus oocytes". *Science* **241** (4867): 835–7.

8. Stephenson FA (November 2006). "Structure and trafficking of NMDA and GABAA receptors". *Biochem. Soc. Trans.* **34** (Pt 5): 877–81. .

9. Teng H. J., Cai W.S., Zhou L.L, Zhang J., Liu Q., Wang Y.Q., Dai W., Zhao M., Sun Z.S. et al. (2010). Desalle, Robert, ed.

"Evolutionary Mode and Functional Divergence of Vertebrate NMDA Receptor Subunit 2 Genes". *PLoS ONE* **5** (10): e13342.

10. Ryan, T. J. & Grant, S. G. N. (2009) The origin and evolution of synapses (vol 10, pg 701, 2009). *Nat Rev Neurosci* 10, Doi 10.1038/Nrn2748

11. Liu XB, Murray KD, Jones EG (October 2004). "Switching of NMDA receptor 2A and 2B subunits at thalamic and cortical synapses during early postnatal development". *J. Neurosci.* **24** (40): 8885–95.

12. Liu Y, Wong TP, Aarts M, Rooyakkers A, Liu L, Lai TW, Wu DC, Lu J, Tymianski M, Craig AM, Wang YT (March 2007). "NMDA receptor subunits have differential roles in mediating excitotoxic neuronal death both in vitro and in vivo". *J. Neurosci.* **27** (11): 2846–57

13. Zhou M, Baudry M (March 2006). "Developmental changes in NMDA neurotoxicity reflect developmental changes in subunit composition of NMDA receptors". *J. Neurosci.* **26** (11): 2956–

14. Sprengel R. et al. (1998). "Importance of the intracellular domain of NR2 subunits for NMDA receptor function in vivo". *Cell* **92** (2): 279–289.

15. Singelyn FJ, Deyaert M, Joris D, (1998): Effects of intravenous patient-controlled analgesia with morphine, continuous epidural analgesia, and continuous three-in-one block on postoperative pain and knee rehabilitation after unilateral total knee arthroplasty. Anesth Analg ; 87: 88–92.

16. Horlocker TT, Cabanela ME, Wedel DJ (1994): Does postoperative epidural analgesia increase the risk of peroneal nerve palsy after total knee arthroplasty? Anesth Analg ; 79: 495–500.

17. Horlocker TT, Wedel D (1998): Neuraxial block and low-molecular-weight heparin: balancing perioperative analgesia and thrombo-prophylaxis. Reg Anesth Pain Med ; 23(6 suppl 2): 164–177.

18. Horlocker TT, Hebl JR, Kinney MA, (2002) : Opioid-free analgesia following total knee arthroplasty—a multimodal approach using continuous lumbar plexus (psoas compartment) block, acetaminophen, and ketorolac. Reg Anesth Pain Med ;27: 105–108.

19. Wheeler M, Oderda GM, Ashburn MA(2002), : Adverse events associated with postoperative opioid analgesia: a systematic review. J Pain ; 3: 159–180.

20. DeWeese FT, Akbari Z, Carline E (2001): Pain control after knee arthroplasty: intra-articular versus epidural anesthesia. Clin Orthop Relat Res ; 392: 226–231.

21. Busch CA, Shore BJ, Bhandari R (1998), : Efficacy of periarticular multimodal drug injection in total knee arthroplasty. A randomized trial. J Bone Joint Surg Am ; 88: 959–963.

22. Koinig H, Wallner T, Marhofer P (1998), : Magnesium sulfate reduces intra- and postoperative analgesic requirements. Anesth Analg ; 87: 206–210.

23. Levaux C, Bonhomme V, Dewandre PY (2003), : Effect of intra-operative magnesium sulphate on pain relief and patient comfort after major lumbar orthopaedic surgery. Anaesthesia ; 58: 131–135.

24. Woolf CJ, Thompson SW(1991): The induction and maintenance of central sensitization is dependent on N-methyl-D-aspartic acid

receptor activation: implications for the treatment of post-injury pain hypersensitivity states. Pain; 44: 293–299.

25.Lawand NB, Willis WD,Westlund K (1997): Excitatory amino acid receptor involvement in peripheral nociceptive transmission in rats. Eur J Pharmacol ;324: 169–177.

26.Cairns BE, Svensson P, Wang K(2003): Activation of peripheral NMDA receptors contributes to human pain and rat afferent discharges evoked by injection of glutamate into the masseter muscle. J Neurophysiol ; 90: 2098–2105.

27.Petrenko AB, Yamakura T,Baba H, (2003) : The role of N-methyl-D-aspartate (NMDA) receptors in pain: a review. Anesth Analg ; 97: 110

28.Kroin JS, McCarthy RJ, Von Roenn N, (1994) : Magnesium sulfate potentiates morphine antinociception at the spinal level. Anesth Analg ; 90: 913–917.Xiao W, Bennett G ,(2000) :Magnesium suppressed neuropathic pain response in rats via spinal site of action. Brain Res ; 666: 168–172.

29.Tramer MR, Schneider J, Marti RA, : Role of magnesium sulphate in postoperative analgesia. Anesthesiology 1996; 84: 340–347.

30.Koinig H, Wallner T, Marhofer P, (1998) : Magnesium sulfate reduces intra- and postoperative analgesic requirements. Anesth Analg ; 87: 206–210.

31.Buvanendran A, Kroin J (2007): Useful adjuvants for postoperative pain management. Best Pract Res Clin Anaesthesiol ; 21: 31–49

32.Thurnau GR, Kemp DB, Jarvis (1987): ACerebrospinal fluid levels of magnesium in patients with preeclampsia after treatment with intravenous magnesium sulfate: a preliminary report. Am J Obstet Gynecol ; 157: 1435–1438.

33. Ascher P, Nowak L (1987): Electrophysiological studies of NMDA receptors. Trends Neurosci ; 10: 284–288

34. Tauzin-Fin P, Sesay M, Svartz L, (2009) : Wound infiltration with magnesium sulphate and ropivacaine mixture reduces postoperative tramadol requirements after radical prostatectomy. Acta Anaesthesiol Scand ; 53: 464–469.

35. Elsharnouby NM, Eid HE, Abou Elezz NF, (2008) : Intraarticular injection of magnesium sulphate and/or bupivacaine for postoperative analgesia after arthroscopic knee surgery. Anesth Analg ; 106: 1548–1552.

36. Yu XM, Sessle BJ, Haas DA, (1996) : Involvement of NMDA receptor mechanisms in jaw electromyographic activity and plasma extravasation induced by irritant application to tempromandibular joint region of rats. Pain ; 68:169–178.

37. 25. Kieffer BL, Evans CJ: Opioid tolerance: In search of the Holy Grail. Cell 2002; 108:587–90 26.

38. Nestler EJ: Molecular basis of long-term plasticity underlying addiction. Nat Rev Neurosci 2001; 2:119–28 27.

39. Nestler EJ, Aghajanian GK: Molecular and cellular basis of addiction. Science 1997; 278:58–63 28.

40. Nestler EJ: Molecular neurobiology of addiction. Am J Addict 2001; 10: 201–17 29.

41. Mao J: Opioid-induced abnormal pain sensitivity: Implications in clinical opioid therapy. Pain 2002; 100:213–7 30.

42. Mayer DJ, Mao J, Holt J, Price DD: Cellular mechanisms of neuropathic pain, morphine tolerance, and their interactions. Proc Natl Acad Sci U S A 1999; 96:7731–6 31.

43. Mao J, Sung B, Ji RR, Lim G: Chronic morphine induces downregulation of spinal glutamate receptors: Implications in morphine tolerance and abnormal pain sensitivity. J Neurosci 2002; 22:8312–23 32.

44. Mao J, Sung B, Ji RR, Lim G: Neuronal apoptosis associated with morphine tolerance: Evidence for an opioid-induced neurotoxic mechanism. J Neurosci 2002; 22:7650–61 33.

45. Vanderah TW, Gardell LR, Burgess SE, Ibrahim M, Dogrul A, Zhang ET, Malan TP, Ossipov MH, Porreca F: Dynorphin promotes abnormal pain and spinal opioid antinociceptive tolerance. J Neurosci 2000; 20:7074–9 34.

46. Basbaum AI: Insights into the development of tolerance. Pain 1995; 61: 349–52 35.

47. Nugent M, Davis C, Brooks D, Ahmedzai SH: Long-term observations of patients receiving transdermal fentanyl after a randomized trial. J Pain Symptom Manage 2001; 21:385–91 36.

48. Fiellin DA, O'Connor PG: Office-based treatment of opioid-dependent patients. N Engl J Med 2002; 347:817–23 37.

49. Fishbain DA, Rosomoff HL, Rosomoff RS: Drug abuse, dependence, and addiction in chronic pain patients. Clin J Pain 1992; 8:77–85 38

50. Doverty M, Somogyi AA, White JM, Bochner F, Beare CH, Menelaou A, Ling W: Methadone maintenance patients are cross-tolerant to the antinociceptive effects of morphine. Pain 2001; 93:155–63 39.

51. Weaver M, Schnoll S: Abuse liability in opioid therapy in pain treatment in patients with an addiction history. Clin J Pain 2002; 18(suppl):S61–9 40.

52. Hoffman M, Povalas A, Lyver A: Pain Management in the opioid addicted patient with cancer. Cancer 1991; 68:1121–3 41.

53. Pasero CL, Compton P: Pain Management in addicted patients. Am J Nursing 1997; 4:17–9 42.

54. Weissman DE, Haddox JD: Opioid pseudoaddiction: An iatrogenic syndrome. Pain 1989; 36:363–6 43.

55. Compton P, Charuvastra VC, Kintaudi K, Ling W: Pain responses in methadone-maintained opioid abusers. J Pain Symptom Manage 2000; 20:237–45 44.

56. Rapp SE, Ready LB, Nessly ML: Acute pain management in patients with prior opioid consumption: A case-controlled retrospective review. Pain 1995; 61:195–201 45.

57. Laulin JP, Celerier E, Larcher A, LeMoal M, Simmonet G: Opiate tolerance to daily heroin administration: An apparent phenomenon associated with enhanced pain sensitivity. Neuroscience 1999; 89:631–6 46.

58. Portenoy RK, Dole V, Joseph H, Lowinson J, Rice C, Segal S, Richman BL: Pain management and chemical dependency: Evolving perspectives. JAMA 1997; 278:592–3 47.

59. Heit HA: The truth about pain management: The difference between a pain patient and an addicted patient. Eur J Pain 2001; 5(suppl A):27–9 48.

60. Sapira JD: The narcotic addict as a medical patient. Am J Med 1968; 45:555–88 49.

61.Robinson RC, Gatchel RJ, Polatin P, Deschner M, Noe C, Gajraj N: Screening for problematic prescription opioid use. Clin J Pain 2001; 17:220–8 50.

62.Kosten TR, Rounsaville BJ, Kleber HD: Antecedents and consequences of cocaine abuse among opioid addicts: A 2.5 year follow-up. J Nerv Ment Dis 1988; 176:176–81 51.

63. Clark HW, Sees KL: Opioids, chronic pain, and the law. J Pain Symptom Manage 1993; 8:297–305 52.

64.Aronoff GM: Opioids in chronic pain management: Is there a significant risk of addiction? Curr Rev Pain 2000; 4:112–21 53

65.Kirsh KL, Whitcomb LA, Donaghy K, Passik SD: Abuse and addiction issues in medically ill patients with pain: Attempts at clarification of terms and empirical study. Clin J Pain 2002; 18(suppl):S52–60 5

66.Savage SR: Assessment for addiction in pain-treatment settings. Clin J Pain 2002; 18(suppl):S28–38 55.

67. Dunbar SA, Katz NP: Chronic opioid therapy for nonmalignant pain in patients with a history of substance abuse: Report of 20 cases. J Pain Symptom Manage 1996; 11:163–71 56.

68.Portenoy RK: Opioid therapy for chronic non-malignant pain: Current status, Progress in Pain Research and Management. Vol 1. Edited by Fields HL, Liebeskind JC. Seattle, IASP, 1994, pp 247–87 57.

69. Chabal C, Erjavec MK, Jacobson L, Mariano A, Chaney E: Prescription opiate abuse in chronic pain patients: Clinical criteria, incidence, and predictors. Clin J Pain 1997; 13:150–5 58.

70.Compton P, Darakjian J, Miotto K: Screening for addiction in patients with chronic pain and "problematic" substance use: Evaluation of a pilot assessment tool. J Pain Symptom Manage 1998; 16:355–63 59.

71. Kreek MJ: Long-term pharmacotherapy for opiate (primarily heroin) addiction: Opioid agonists, Handbook of Experimental Pharmacology. Opioids II. Vol 118. Edited by Schuster CR, Kuhar MJ. New York, Springer Verlag, 1996, pp 487–562 60.

72. Rubenstein RB, Spira I, Wolff WI: Management of surgical problems in patients of methadone maintenance. Am J Surgery 1976; 131:566–9 61.

73.Johnson RE, Jaffe JH, Fudala PJ: A controlled trial of buprenorphine treatment for opioid dependence. JAMA 1992; 287:2750–5 6

74.Reuben SS, Connelly NR: Postoperative analgesic effects of celecoxib or rofecoxib after spinal fusion surgery. Anesth Analg 2000; 91:1221–5 63.

75. Sevarino FB, Ning T: Transdermal fentanyl for acute pain management, Acute Pain: Mechanisms and Management. Edited by Sinatra RS, Hord AH, Ginsberg B, Preble LM. St. Louis, Missouri, Mosby Yearbook, 1992, pp 364–9 64.

76. Caplan RA, Ready B, Oden RV, Matsen FA, Nessly ML, Olsson GL: Transdermal fentanyl for postoperative pain management. JAMA 1989; 261:1036–9 65.

77.Patt RB: PCA: Prescribing analgesia for home management of severe pain. Geriatrics 1992; 47:69–72 66.

78.Gomar C, Carrero EJ: Delayed arousal after general anesthesia associated with baclofen. ANESTHESIOLOGY 1994; 81:1306–7 67.

79. Foley RM: Opioid analgesics in clinical pain management, Handbook of Experimental Pharmacology. Opioids II. Vol 104. Edited by Herz A, Akil H, Simon EJ. New York, Springer Verlag, 1993, pp 697–743 68.

80. Reisine T, Pasternak G: Opioid analgesics and antagonists, Goodman and Gilman's The Pharmacological Basis of Therapeutics, 9th edition. Edited by Hardman JG, Limbird LE, Molinoff PB, Ruddon RW, Gilman AG. New York, McGraw-Hill, 1996, pp 521–55 69.

81. Manfredi PL, Ribeiro S, Cahndler SW, Payne R: Inappropriate use of naloxone in cancer patients with pain. J Pain Symptom Manage 1996; 11:131–4 70.

82. Thomas AN, Suresh M: Opiate withdrawal after tramadol and PCA (letter). Anaesthesia 2000; 53:826–7 71.

83. Gonzales JP, Brogden RN: Naltrexone: A review of its pharmacodynamic and pharmacokinetic properties and therapeutic efficacy in the treatment of opioid dependence. Drugs 1988; 35:192–213 72.

84. Saberski L: Postoperative pain management for the patient with chronic pain, Acute Pain: Mechanisms and Management. Edited by Sinatra RS, Hord AH, Ginsb Groc L, Choquet D, Stephenson FA, Verrier D, Manzoni OJ, Chavis P (2007). "NMDA receptor surface trafficking and synaptic subunit composition are developmentally regulated by the extracellular matrix protein Reelin". *J. Neurosci.* **27** (38): 10165–75.

85. Espinosa JS, Luo LJ (March 2008). "Timing neurogenesis and differentiation: insights from quantitative clonal analyses of cerebellar granule cells". *J. Neurosci.* **28** (10): 2301

86. Gajendran N, Kapfhammer JP, Lain E, Canepari M, Vogt K, Wisden W, Brenner HR (February 2009). "Neuregulin Signaling Is Dispensable for NMDA- and GABAA-Receptor Expression in the Cerebellum In Vivo". *J. Neurosci.* **29** (8): 2404–13..

87. Chen PE, Geballe MT, Stansfeld PJ, Johnston AR, Yuan H, Jacob AL, Snyder JP, Traynelis SF, Wyllie DJ (May 2005). "Structural features of the glutamate binding site in recombinant NR1/NR2A N-methyl-D-aspartate receptors determined by site-directed mutagenesis and molecular modeling". *Mol. Pharmacol.* **67** (5): 1470–84.

88. Wolosker H (Oct 2006). "D-serine regulation of NMDA receptor activity". *Sci. STKE* **pe41**(356): 1–3.

89. Yarotskyy V, Glushakov AV, Sumners C, Gravenstein N, Dennis DM, Seubert CN, Martynyuk AE (May 2005). "Differential modulation of glutamatergic transmission by 3,5-dibromo-L-phenylalanine". *Mol. Pharmacol.* **67** (5): 1648–54.

90. Moskal, D. Leander, R. Burch (2010). Unlocking the Therapeutic Potential of the NMDA Receptor. *Drug Discovery & Development News.* Retrieved 19 December 2013.

91. Anderson C (2003-06-01). "The Bad News Isn't In: A Look at Dissociative-Induced Brain Damage and Cognitive Impairment". *Erowid DXM Vaults : Health.* Retrieved 2008-12-17.

92. "Effects of N-Methyl-D-Aspartate (NMDA)-Receptor Antagonism on Hyperalgesia, Opioid Use, and Pain After Radical Prostatectomy". ClinicalTrials.gov. 2005-09-01. Retrieved2008-12-17.

93. "Atomoxetine acts as an NMDA receptor blocker in clinically relevant concentrations". British Journal of Pharmacology. 2013-05-08. Retrieved 2010-03-02.

94. Huggins DJ, Grant GH (January 2005). "The function of the amino terminal domain in NMDA receptor modulation". *J. Mol. Graph. Model.* **23** (4): 8.

95. Traynelis, Stephen; Cull-Candy (May 24, 1990)Stuart". *Nature* **345** (6273):50.

96. Aizenman E, Lipton SA, Loring RH (March 1989). "Selective modulation of NMDA responses by reduction and oxidation". *Neuron* **2** (3): 1257

97. Yu XM, Askalan R, Keil GJ, Salter MW (January 1997). "NMDA channel regulation by channel-associated protein tyrosine kinase Src". *Science* **275** (5300): 674–8.

98. Chen Y, Beffert U, Ertunc M, Tang TS, Kavalali ET, Bezprozvanny I, Herz J (September 2005). "Reelin modulates NMDA receptor activity in cortical neurons". *J. Neurosci.* **25**(36): 8209–16

99. Hawasli AH, Benavides DR, Nguyen C, Kansy JW, Hayashi K, Chambon P, Greengard P, Powell CM, Cooper DC, Bibb JA (July 2007). "Cyclin-dependent kinase 5 governs learning and synaptic plasticity via control of NMDAR degradation". *Nat. Neurosci.* **10** (7): 880–6.

100.   Zhang S, Edelmann L, Liu J, Crandall JE, Morabito MA (January 2008). "Cdk5 regulates the phosphorylation of tyrosine 1472 NR2B and the surface expression of NMDA receptors". *J. Neurosci.* **28** (2): 415–24.

101.   Fourgeaud L, Davenport CM, Tyler CM, Cheng TT, Spencer MB, Boulanger LM (December 2010). "MHC class I modulates NMDA receptor function and AMPA receptor trafficking". *Proc Natl Acad Sci U S A* **107** (51): 22278–83.

102.   Huh GS, Boulanger LM, Du H, Riquelme PA, Brotz TM, Shatz CJ (December 2000)."Functional requirement for class I MHC in CNS development and plasticity". *Science***290** (5499): 2155–9. .

103.   Nelson, PA; Sage, JR; Wood, SC; Davenport, CM; Anagnostaras, SG; Boulanger, LM (Sep 1, 2013). "MHC class I immune proteins are critical for hippocampus-dependent memory and gate NMDAR-dependent hippocampal long-term depression.". *Learning & memory (Cold Spring Harbor, N.Y.)* **20** (9): 505–17.

104.   Purves, Dale; George J. Augustine, David Fitzpatrick, William C. Hall, Anthony-Samuel LaMantia, James O. McNamara, Leonard E. White (2008). *Neuroscience, 4th Ed.*Sinauer Associates. pp. 129–131. ISBN 978-0-87893-697-7.

105.   Purves, Dale; George J. Augustine, David Fitzpatrick, William C. Hall, Anthony-Samuel LaMantia, James O. McNamara, Leonard E. White (2008). *Neuroscience, 4th Ed.*Sinauer Associates. pp. 191–195. ISBN 978-0-87893-697-7

106.   Mount C, Downton C (July 2006). "Alzheimer disease: progress or profit?". *Nat Med.* **12**(7): 780–4. doi:10.1038/nm0706-780. PMID 16829947.

107.   NICE technology appraisal January 18, 2011 Azheimer's disease - donepezil, galantamine, rivastigmine and memantine (review): final appraisal determination

108.   Wijesinghe, R (2014). "Emerging Therapies for Treatment Resistant Depression". *Ment Health Clin* **4** (5): 56. ISSN 2168-9709.

109.   Linda Poon (2014). "Growing Evidence That A Party Drug Can Help Severe Depression". NPR.

110.   Gary Stix (2014). "From Club to Clinic: Physicians Push Off-Label Ketamine as Rapid Depression Treatment". Scientific American.

111.   Lisman JE, Coyle JT, Green RW et al. (May 2008). "Circuit-based framework for understanding neurotransmitter and risk gene interactions in schizophrenia". *Trends in Neurosciences* **31** (5): 234–42. doi:10.1016/j.tins.2008.02.005. PMC 2680493.PMID 18395805.

112.   Liu XB, Murray KD, Jones EG (October 2004). "Switching of NMDA receptor 2A and 2B subunits at thalamic and cortical synapses during early postnatal development". *J. Neurosci.* **24** (40): 8885–95. Actions of Bupivacaine, a Widely Used Local Anesthetic, on NMDA Receptor Response

113.   M. Schley, S. Topfner, K. Wiech,H.E. Schaller, C.J. Konrad[1], M.Schmelz[1]andN. Birbaumer[2,4]Continuous brachial plexus blockade in combination with the NMDA receptor antagonist memantine prevents phantom pain in acute traumatic upper limb amputees Article first published online: 9 JAN 2012 2007 European Federation of Chapters of the International Association for the Study of Painm.Low SJ, Roland CLInt J Clin Pharmacol Ther. 2004 Jan;42(1):1-14.

114.   Wijesinghe, R (2014). "Emerging Therapies for Treatment Resistant Depression". *Ment Health Clin* **4** (5): 56. ISSN 2168-9709.

115.   Himmelseher, S.; Pfenninger, E. (2008). "Die klinische Anwendung von S-(+)-Ketamin - eine Standortbestimmung". *AINS - Anästhesiologie · Intensivmedizin · Notfallmedizin · Schmerztherapie* **33** (12): 764–770.

116.   Ihmsen, H.; Geisslinger, G.; Schüttler, J. (2001). "Stereoselective pharmacokinetics of ketamine: R(-)-ketamine inhibits the elimination of S(+)-ketamine". *Clinical pharmacology and therapeutics* **70** (5): 431–438. doi:10.1067/mcp.2001.119722.PMID 11719729. edit

117.   Nishimura, M.; Sato, K. (1999). "Ketamine stereoselectively inhibits rat dopamine transporter". *Neuroscience letters* **274** (2): 131–134.

118.   Doenicke, A.; Kugler, J.; Mayer, M.; Angster, R.; Hoffmann, P. (1992). "Ketamine racemate or S-(+)-ketamine and midazolam. The effect on vigilance, efficacy and subjective findings". *Der Anaesthesist* **41** (10): 610–618.

119.   Pfenninger, E.; Baier, C.; Claus, S.; Hege, G. (1994). "Psychometric changes as well as analgesic action and cardiovascular adverse effects of ketamine racemate versus s-(+)-ketamine in subanesthetic doses". *Der Anaesthesist.* 43 Suppl 2: S68–S75.

120.   Vollenweider, F. X.; Leenders, K. L.; Oye, I.; Hell, D.; Angst, J. (1997). "Differential psychopathology and patterns of cerebral glucose utilisation produced by (S)- and (R)-ketamine in healthy volunteers using positron emission tomography (PET)". *European neuropsychopharmacology : the journal of the European College of Neuropsychopharmacology* **7** (1): 25–3

121.   Zhang, J. C.; Li, S. X.; Hashimoto, K. (2014). "R (−)-ketamine shows greater potency and longer lasting antidepressant effects than S (+)-ketamine". *Pharmacology Biochemistry and Behavior* **116**: 137–141.

122.   Carboni E, Tanda GL, Frau R, Di Chiara G (1990). "Blockade of the noradrenaline carrier increases extracellular dopamine concentrations in the prefrontal cortex: evidence that dopamine is taken up in vivo by noradrenergic terminals". *J. Neurochem.* **55** (3): 1067–70.

123.   **Effects of S-ketamine as an anesthetic adjuvant to propofol on treatment response to electroconvulsive therapy in treatment-resistant depression: a randomized pilot study.**

124.   Järventausta K[1], Chrapek W, Kampman O, Tuohimaa K, Björkqvist M, Häkkinen H, Yli-Hankala A, Leinonen E.Pain Physician. 2010 Jul-Aug;13(4):365-8.

125.   The use of sub-anesthetic intravenous ketamine and adjuvant dexmedetomidine when treating acute pain from CRPS.Nama S[1], Meenan DR, Fritz WT.J Pediatr Hematol Oncol. 2004 Oct;26(10):678-80.

126.   Tsui BC[1], Davies D, Desai S, Malherbe S Intravenous ketamine infusion as an adjuvant to morphine in a 2-year-old with severe cancer pain from metastatic neuroblastoma. J Pediatr Hematol Oncol. 2004 Oct;26(10):678-80.

Intra peritoneal S Ketamine reduces postoperative analgesic requirements in morbidly obese patients a controlled study.

Hala Mostafa Goma ;MD,

Corresponding author: Hala Mostafa Goma, assistant professor of anesthesia, Cairo university.

E-mail ahmeda1995@yahoo.com

Abstract:

Background: this study was designed to evaluate the role of intraperitoneal S (+) ketamine in peripheral NMDA receptors blockade, and whether it reduces the postoperative analgesic requirements after bariatric surgery in morbidly obese patients in comparison with intraperitoneal lidocaine.

Patients and methods:

The study included 45 patients, and a standardized general anesthetic technique including fentanyl, propofol, isoflurane, and vecuronium for muscle relaxation were used. At the end of surgery, patients were divided into three groups ,15 patients each, S (+) Ketamine 0.5 mg /kg diluted in 50 ml saline was injected intra peritoneally in (ketamine group), 50 ml of 1% lidocaine in saline was injected intra peritoneally in (lidocaine group), 50 ml of normal saline was injected intra peritoneally in (saline group). Parameters were evaluated time of first request of analgesia in minutes ,postoperative shoulder pain and arm pain for 24 hours(VAS score), and the amount of post operative mepridine (mg) consumed in 0-6.6-12,12-18,18-24,hours after extubation.

Results: Times of the first request of postoperative analgesia were 60(10), 50(5), 20(5) minutes, in Intra peritoneal S Ketamine group, Intra peritoneal lidocaine group, and Intra peritoneal Saline group respectively. It was statistically longer in Ketamine group and Lidocaine group than Saline group, with statistically longer duration in Ketamine group than Lidocaine group.

However the amount of mepridine was statistically higher in Lidocaine group and Saline group than in Ketamine group, at 6, 8,12,18,24 hours postoperatively, it was statistically higher in Saline group than in Lidocaine group.

Both the incidence postoperative shoulder pain, and the visual analogue score were significantly higher in Lidocaine group and Saline group than in Ketamine group, but it was statistically higher in Saline group than in Lidocaine group.

Conclusion:

Peripheral (peritoneal) NMDA receptors blockade by S (+) Ketamine was involved in reduction of postoperative pain, and analgesic requirement following bariatric surgery.

Key words: intraperitoneal, S Ketamine, morbidly obese.

Introduction:

Bariatric surgery at the upper extremes of weight can be associated with serious postoperative complications (Helling et al 2004) the complication are postoperative hypoventilation, hypoxia, hypercapnia, and postoperative pain (Gasynski et al 2007) . The incidence of postoperative shoulder pain following laparoscopic surgery may reach up to 80% (Collins KM et al 1984), and it represents a major cause for high unanticipated admission rate up to 12.1 % (Hedayati and Fear 1999).

Experimentally, intra peritoneal administration of NMDA receptor antagonists decreased the nociception observed during the late phase of the formalin test (Berrino et al 2003). Animal studies have shown that S ketamine has approximately four times more affinity for phencyclidine binding area in NMDA receptors as compared to (R -) ketamine (Mc Cartehy et al 2004) . Increased affinity for the receptor ,combined with similar pharmacokinetics suggests that S (+)ketamine could be clinically interesting drug (Taura et al 2003),in rats and mice S(+) ketamine has 1.5-3 times higher hypnotic potency and 3 times higher analgesic potency as compared with – ketamine being twice more potent than racemic mixture (Koga et al 1994) .

Aim of this study was to assess the analgesic effects of intra peritoneal ketamine S (+) (NMDA receptors antagonist), and compare its analgesic effect with intra peritoneal 0.1 % Lidocaine.

Patients and methods:

The study include 45 morbidly obese patients (BMI>40) ,ASA I,II admitted to surgical ICU in new Kasr El Ani Hospital ,after laparoscopic bariatric surgery with absence of primary cardiac or chest disease. After the approval of ethics committee, written   consents from patients preoperatively were taken.

Patients were divided into 3 groups, 15 patients each , the first group was S (+)ketamine group(K group), the second group was lidocaine group(L group) and the third group was normal saline group(S group).

Exclusion criteria: Were Cardiac disease, Diabetes mellitus, Gross anemia, hemoglobinopathies, polycythemia, Hepatic disease, Ischemic cerebrovascular disease, renal disease, Respiratory insufficiency, severe systemic hypertension.

For premedication midazolam 0.05 mg/kg IV was given 15 minute before induction.

 Induction of anesthesia was achieved by 2.5-3 mg /kg propofol injected intravenously on 3-5 minute to prevent sudden drop of blood pressure, fentanyl 1μg/kg iv. Tracheal intubation with cuffed endotracheal tube was facilitated with 0.1mg/kg vecuronium. Nasogastric tube was inserted.

Maintenance of anesthesia:

Anesthesia was maintained with 50% O_2 in air with 1.3 MAC of isoflurane, and then 0.05 mg/Kg vecuronium.

 Ventilation was adjusted to maintain end tidal CO_2 between 30-35mmHg

 6 ml/kg/hour IV crystalloid solution was given,

Monitoring included non invasive blood pressure measurement, SO2 (O2 saturation), end tidal CO2, and ECG.

A small about 1 cm elliptical sub umbilical incision was used to introduce the Vress needle towards the pelvis with patients in the Trendelenburg position. pneumoperitoneum was achieved by insufflation of CO2at rate 1 L /min for the first minute, then at rate of 3-4 L/minute with a maximum intra-abdominal pressure of 15 mmHg. Introduction of a safety reusable metal trocar through the previous incision was done .The camera scope was then introduced and the pelvis was inspected for any site of bleeding .Patients were put in anti- Trendelenburg position with rising of the right shoulder. At the end of the surgical procedure, patients were randomly allocated into one of the three equal groups. In (K group) S (+) Ketamine 0.5 mg /kg diluted in 50 ml saline was injected intra peritoneally, in (L group) 50 ml 1% lidocaine in saline was injected, in S group 50 ml of normal saline was injected intra peritoneally. In the three studied groups, intra peritoneal injection was guided by camera under both copulae of the diaphragm, and patients kept in the Trendelenburg position till the end of intraperitoneal injection (10-15 minute). Pain was assessed using Visual Analogue Scale (VAS), where zero score corresponds to no pain. All patients were admitted to postoperative surgical ICU, where they were monitored by O2 saturation, ECG, blood pressure. CPAP of 5- 10 cm H2O was used via face mask.

Post operative pain was initially managed with bolus of 0.5 mg /kg IV mepridine and increased gradually to 1 mg/kg IV mepridine if there was inadequate analgesia, (VAS) was repeated every 6 hours for the first 24 hours, mepridine was given in a dose of 0.25 mg IV, and it was increased gradually after 15 minutes if there was in adequate analgesia. The following parameters were evaluated in all studied groups:

1. Time of first request of analgesia (time elapsed from extubation to the first analgesic dose).

2.the amount of postoperative mepridine was consumed in 0-6 h,6-12 h,12-18 h,18-24h,,and 0-24 following extubation.

3. The incidence and severity of postoperative shoulder pain for 24 hours, it represents the mean of pain scores measured at 0-6, 6-12, 12-18, and 18-24 hours postoperatively.

Statistical analysis:

Data are expressed as mean and (SD). One way ANOVA was used to detect both time to first request of analgesia and the variability in the VAS in between the studied groups, with post hoc Newman-Keules test. Chi-squared or Fisher exact test were used, as appropriate, to compare incidences of side effects and postoperative pain in different groups. All significant results were carried out the 5% level.

Table (1): patients and operative data .values are mean (SD).

	K group (n=15)	L group (n=15)	S group (n=15)
Age (years)	24 ,1(6.5)	23(7.4)	22 .2 (8.1)
Sex (male /female)	8/7	9/6	7/8
Weight (kg)	130(25)	128(26)	126(27)
Height (cm)	170(10)	169(11)	168(12)
BMI(kg/m^2)	43 (1.9)	42(2.7)	42 (2.8)
ASAI/II	10/5	11/4	12/3
Duration of surgery(minutes)	120(25)	125(20)	122(22)

K group = Intra peritoneal S (+) ketamine group; L group = Intra peritoneal lidocaine group, S group = Intra peritoneal saline group.

Table 2: post operative analgesic requirements, time to first request of analgesia, incidence, and severity of post operative shoulder pain. Values are means (SD) or number and percent % of patients.

	K group (n=15)	L group (n=15)	S group (n=15)
Time to first request of postoperative mepridine (min)	60(10)	50(5) *	20(5)* †
Dose of mepridine (mg)			
0-6 h	80 (5.3)	120(12.2) *	150 (8.2) *†
6-12h	60 (4.5)	100(10.4) *	130 (5.4) *†
12 -18h	40 (5.4)	85 (15.3) *	100 (10.1) *†
18-24h	25 (3.5)	60 (5.2) *	80 (7.5) *†
0-24h	205 (4.6)	365(10.3) *	460 (7.8) *†
Incidence % of postoperative shoulder pain	3 (20%)	7(46.7%)*	12 (80%)*†
Visual analogue shoulder pain score	2 (0.4)	4(0.9) *	6.4(0.6) *†

K Group = Ketamine S (+) group; L group =lidocaine group; S group= normal saline group.

* Comparison was between the three groups.

†comparison was between lidocaine group (L group), and saline group (S group).

Results:

Patient's characteristics and operative details were comparable among the three groups (table 1).

Times of the first request of postoperative analgesia were 60(10), 50(5), 20(5) minutes, in Intra peritoneal S (+) Ketamine group (K group), Intra peritoneal lidocaine group (L group), and Intra peritoneal Saline group (S group) respectively. It was statistically longer in K group and L group than S group, with statistically longer duration in K group than L group table 2.

However the amount of mepridine was statistically higher in group L, and group S than in group K, at 6, 8,12,18,24 hours postoperatively, it was statistically higher in group S than group L table 2.

Both the incidence postoperative shoulder pain, and the visual analogue score were significantly higher in group L and group S than group K, but it was statistically higher in group S than in group L table 2.

Discussion:

The present study demonstrated that intra peritoneal S (+) ketamine was associated with reduction of both postoperative shoulder pain, and the analgesic requirements in patients underwent laparoscopic bariatric surgery. The efficacy of intra peritoneal Ketamine S (+) was superior to the intra peritoneal lidocaine .N-methyl –D-aspartate (NMDA)receptor activation is considered one of the mechanism of postoperative pain, and the hypersensitivity through both peripheral (intraperitoneal) ,and central effects (intravenous route) (Wilder-Smith et al1997) . Peripheral NMDA receptors are important in normal visceral pain transmission, and may provide a noval mechanism for development of peripheral sanitization, and visceral hyperalgesia (McRoberts et al 2001). At the same time, N-methyl-D aspartate (NMDA) activation plays an important role in wind up. Activation of NMDA receptors increases intracellular calcium concentration in spinal neurons and activates both phospholipase C (PLC), and phospholipase A2 (PLA2), activation of NMDA receptors also induces nitric oxide synthetase, resulting in formation of nitric oxide (NO). Both prostaglandin and nitric oxide facilitate the release of excitatory amino acids in the spinal cord (Carlton et al 1999). In the present study intra peritoneal Ketamine S (+) reduced postoperative shoulder pain, and reduced the total dose of required mepridine, this could be explained by peripheral blockade of peripheral NMDA receptors. Many studies observed the role of intra peritoneal NMDA receptors blockade (Berrino et al 2003) demonstrated the anti nociceptive effects in mice of intra peritoneal N methyl –D aspartate receptor antagonists in the formalin test.

Davidson et al (1997) demonstrated that peripheral NMDA and non NMDA glutamate receptor contribute to nociceptive behavior in the rat formalin test. **Nadeson et al** (2002) concluded that S (+) **ketamine** can potentiate the effects of fentanyl by an interaction at the level of the spinal cord even when **ketamine** was given via the intra peritoneal route in rats. Borner et al (2007) concluded that the application of intra articular S (+) ketamine (peripheral NMDA receptors antagonism) after arthroscopic knee surgery led to a significant decrease of postoperative analgesic demand.

Conclusion:

Peripheral (peritoneal) NMDA receptors blockade by S (+) Ketamine was involved in reduction of postoperative pain, and analgesic requirement following bariatric surgery.

References:

1. Helling TS, Willoughby TL, Maxfield DM, Ryan P; 2004: Determinants of the need for intensive care and prolonged mechanical ventilation in patients undergoing bariatric surgery. Obes Surg. Sep; 14(8):1036-41.

2. Gaszynski T, Tokarz A, Piotrowski D, Machala W: 2007; Boussignac CPAP in the postoperative period in morbidly obese patients. Obes Surg Apr; 17(4):452-6

3. Hedayati B, Fear S: 1999; Hospital admission after day-case gynaecological laparoscopy. Br J Anaesth. Nov;83(5):776-9

4. Berrino L, Oliva P, Massimo F, Aurilio C, Maione S, Grella A, Rossi F: 2003; Antinociceptive effect in mice of intraperitoneal N-methyl-D-aspartate receptor antagonists in the formalin test. Eur J Pain.; 7(2):131-7.

5. Mc Cartehy C,A.Shinha,and Jkatz,2004:A qualitative systemic review of the role of N-methyl aspartate receptors antagonists in preventive analgesia .anesthesia Analg.98:1385-1400.

6. Taurá P, Fuster J, Blasi A, Martinez-Ocon J, Anglada T, Beltran J, Balust J, Tercero J, Garcia-Valdecasas JC. 2003: Postoperative pain relief after hepatic resection in cirrhotic patients: the efficacy of a single small dose of ketamine plus morphine epidurally. Anesth Analg. Feb; 96(2):475-80, table of contents

7. Takenaka I, Ogata M, Koga K, Matsumoto T, Shigematsu A;1994 :Ketamine suppresses endotoxin-induced tumor necrosis factor alpha production in mice. Anesthesiology. Feb; 80(2):402-8.

8.Wilder-Smith CH, Knöpfli R, Wilder-Smith OH: 1997 ,Perioperative magnesium infusion and postoperative pain Acta Anaesthesiol Scand. Sep;41(8):1023-7.

9.McRoberts JA, Coutinho SV, Marvizón JC, Grady EF, Tognetto M, Sengupta JN, Ennes HS, Chaban VV, Amadesi S, Creminon C, Lanthorn T, Geppetti P, Bunnett NW, Mayer EA: 2001: Role of peripheral N-methyl-D-aspartate (NMDA) receptors in visceral nociception in rats. Gastroenterology. Jun; 120(7):1737-48.

10.Carlton SM, Zhou S, Coggeshall RE; 1999: Peripheral GABA(A) receptors , evidence for peripheral primary afferent depolarization. Neuroscience.; 93(2):713-22

11.Berrino L, Oliva P, Massimo F, Aurilio C, Maione S, Grella A, Rossi F; 2003 : Antinociceptive effect in mice of intraperitoneal N-methyl-D-aspartate receptor antagonists in the formalin test. Eur J Pain.; 7(2):131-7.

12.Davidson EM, Coggeshall RE, Carlton SM: 1997, Peripheral NMDA andnon-NMDA glutamate receptors contribute to nociceptive behaviors in the rat formalin test. Neuroreport. Mar 3;8(4):941-6.

13.Borner M, Bürkle H, Trojan S, Horoshun G, Riewendt HD, Wappler F. 2007: [Intra-articular ketamine after arthroscopic knee surgery. Optimisation of postoperative analgesia] Anaesthesist. Nov; 56(11):1120-7.

Research article

Effect of single versus repeated doses of intravenous S (+) ketamine on the release of proinflammatory cytokines in patients undergoing radical prostatectomy.

Author HALA Mostafa Goma,MD

Professor of anesthesia , Faculty of medicine ,Cairo University.

Abstract:

The stimulus of surgery leads to increase in the concentrations of proinflammatory cytokines and altered immune response (1). Proinflammatory cytokines modulate pain indirectly through the release of certain substances like nitric oxide, oxygen free radicals and prostaglandins leading to peripheral and central sensitivity and hyperalgesia (2). Excessive production of proinflammatory cytokines due to anesthesia and surgical trauma may provoke severe inflammatory response and post-operative complications (3). Thus if there is a drug that may be used to decrease the level of proinflammatory cytokines we may achieve more favorable postoperative outcome. Cytokines are low molecular weight proteins which after binding to specific receptors affect immune cell differentiation, proliferation, and activity. Proinflammatory cytokines comprise number of factors like tumor necrosis factor alpha, interleukin 6 and interleukin 8. The rationale of the study was to evaluate the role of S (+) ketamine in decreasing the unwanted effect of anesthesia and surgery on the immune system (4).

Patients and methods: This study was a prospective randomized controlled double-blinded trial. After approval of local ethical committee, informed written consent was obtained from all patients, 60 patients ASA physical status I–III, aged over 45 years old scheduled for radical prostatectomy under combined epidural general anesthesia in Urology Theater in Cairo University teaching hospital were included in this study. Exclusion criteria were ; ASA physical status > III, morbid obesity (body mass index > 35), pre-existing neurological or psychiatric disorders, chronic drug abuse, the use of drugs affecting immunity as chemotherapy or hormonal therapy, uncontrolled diabetics, renal, hepatic, hypertensive patients, contraindication for epidural catheter insertion, hypersensitivity for any anesthetics or drug used. Patients were randomly divided into 3groups according to randomized sequences without duplicates, 20 patients in each group. Group I: received combined epidural-general anesthesia without S (+) ketamine (control group), Group II: received combined epidural-general anesthesia and S (+) ketamine as a single preincision dose, Group III: received combined epidural-general anesthesia and S (+) ketamine as preincision and repeated doses up to 4 hours of surgery. In the preparation room under local anesthesia intravenous cannula was inserted, midazolam 1 mg and ranitidine 50 mg were given to all patients. Then the patient was transferred to the operating room, standard monitors were applied, then epidural catheter was inserted under complete aseptic technique to supplement general anesthesia and to control postoperative pain. Then general anesthesia was induced with propofol (2 mg/kg), fentanyl (1μg/kg) and atracurium 0.5 mg/kg to facilitate tracheal intubation. For maintenance of anesthesia an infusion of atracurium at rate of 8μg /kg/min and 1-1.5% isoflurane and 100% O_2 was used, ventilator parameter was adjusted to keep EtCO2 between 30-35 mmHg, 5 ml of levobupivacaine 0.25% was administrated in epidural catheter and repeated according the hemodynamic variables. Blood samples were drawn immediately after induction of anesthesia and before S (+) ketamine injection to determine the baseline of cytokines that were measured (TNF-α and IL-6) then S (+) ketamine (Pfizer, Karlsruhe, Germany) was injected as a single IV dose 0.5 mg/kg before incision in group II and III and repeated 0.2 mg/kg doses at 20 minute intervals till the end of surgery (in group III only). The blood samples were taken after 1 hour in group I and II and hourly after S (+) ketamine injection till four hours of surgery and 1 hour after surgery in group III. Blood was collected on EDTA tubes and centrifuged at 3.000 rpm for 15 minutes. Plasma was stored at -80°C until the moment of analysis. TNF-α and IL-6 levels were measured using The RayBio® Human TNF-alpha ELISA (Enzyme-Linked Immunosorbent Assay) kits. Statistical analyses were performed using SPSS 14.0 (SPSS Inc., Chicago, IL, USA); study data were expressed as mean ± SD and percentage as appropriate. The sample size was calculated based on the hypothesis that the difference in cytokine concentration in the groups that receiving ketamine would be at least 25%. In order to have a 95% chance to detect this difference at a level of significance ($p < 0.05$), the number of patients calculated by group was 18 we added 2 patients for dropouts. A p-value ≤ 0.05 was considered significant.

Results: There was no statistically significant difference between the 3 groups as regarding demographic data (age, gender, weight, ASA physical status and duration of anesthesia). No serious adverse effects were recorded in all groups.

Variable	Group I (n=20)	Group II (n=20)	Group III (n=20)
Age (yr)	44-60	47-62	48-61
Gender (m/f)	13/7	12/8	14/6
Weight (kg)	75-82	74-81	77-80
Duration of anesthesia (min)	280±25	275±30	285±42

Total dose of levobupivacaine was significantly decreased in group II and more in group III this indicates the analgesic effect of S (+) ketamine,

Variable	Group I (n=20)	Group II (n=20)	Group III (n=20)
Total dose of levobupivacaine (mg)	250 mg ± 50 mg	190 mg ± 20 mg	130mg ± 15mg

Serum levels of TNF-α and IL-6 were done for control and treatment groups at 2 different time points (preincision and 1hr later) and the mean TNF-α and mean IL-6 levels were compared among each group separately and showed that: among group (I) patients mean TNF-α and mean IL-6 increased at the 2nd time point and this rise was highly statistically significant for both values *(P<0.001)*; while among group Π and Group Ш mean TNF-α and mean IL-6 decreased at the 2nd time point and this reduction was highly statistically significant *(P<0.001)*.

Comparison of TNF-α and IL-6 at the 1st time point (the preincision) between the 3 study groups showed no significant difference. But comparison of the mean TNF-α and IL-6 at the 2nd time point (1hr later) between the 3 study groups showed that the differences in the mean values among the treatment groups is highly statistically significant *(P<0.001)*

In group III comparison of the TNF-α and IL-6 levels at the different time points (preincision, hourly for 4 hours intraoperatively and 1 hour postoperatively) showed that the TNF-α and IL-6 were significantly decreased throughout the perioperative period compared with the baseline value ***(P<0.001)***

Discussion: Radical prostatectomy is a major surgical procedure associated with marked surgical trauma and release of proinflammatory cytokines. S (+) ketamine was chosen as it has better recovery profile with less hallucination or mood changes, S (+) ketamine; the left handed optical isomer of racemic ketamine, has fourfold higher affinity to NMDA receptors than its isomer R (–) ketamine that approximately twice that of racemic ketamine (5). We found that the total dose of epidural levobupivacaine was reduced in single dose ketamine group and more reduced in multiple dose ketamine group than control group, This study shows the effect of S (+) ketamine in decreasing the level of cytokines, and that leads to less noxious stimulation, less hyperalgesia, and subsequent decrease in the dose of opioid and local anesthetics, This study, also revealed that, when S (+) ketamine used as a single dose before the incision, it decreased the level of cytokines, but when used as repeated intravenous doses the cytokine levels decreased more and there was significant difference between single and repeated doses, the dose of ropivacaine was significantly lower in the repeated doses of S (+) ketamine this results was in agreement of the results of Snijdelaar et al. (6). He found that the low dose of S (+) ketamine given during and after radical prostatectomy reduced PCA morphine consumption by 34% at 48 hours after surgery and lower pain scores at rest compared with standard treatment ; control group, that did not receive S (+) ketamine (6). It is now recognized that the process of central sensitization is induced not only during surgery but also postoperatively by inflammatory injuries (7). In the clinical setting this suggests that for optimal effect of NMDA receptor antagonists need to be administrated before induction of anesthesia and continued during surgery and in the postoperative period (8). Roytblat et al. reported that a single dose of ketamine 0.25 mg/kg administered before cardiopulmonary bypass suppressed the increase in serum IL- 6 during and after coronary artery bypass surgery (9), and that a subanesthetic dose of ketamine suppressed IL-6 production in women undergoing hysterectomy (10).

Ilkjaer et al. investigated the additive analgesic effects of ketamine on postoperative pain after renal surgery, In this study, a bolus dose of ketamine 10 mg, followed by an infusion of ketamine 10 mg/h for 48 hours after operation, was administered IV (11). The authors concluded that ketamine did not reduce postoperative pain and that larger doses of ketamine would provide increased analgesia. Fu et al. showed that 0.5 mg/kg of ketamine had a preemptive analgesic effect in patients undergoing abdominal procedures (12). Tverskoy et al. reported a decrease in wound hyperalgesia for 48 hours after ketamine anesthesia. We believe that this long-lasting postoperative analgesia might be explained with a preemptive analgesic effect of ketamine, but further investigation is necessary to clarify underlying mechanism of this persistent analgesic effect of ketamine (13). Kawasaki and colleagues had carried out in vitro studies with human whole blood and reported a suppressive effect of ketamine on LPS-induced TNF-α, IL-6, and IL-8 production. TNF-α is the first cytokine which stimulates IL-6 and IL-8 production by macrophages (14). Hala Mostafa et al reported a decrease in proinflammatory cytokines in major abdominal surgery under combined general epidural anesthesia.

Conclusion, preincional and repeated use of intraoperative S (+) ketamine as an analgesic adjunct to general and epidural anesthesia improves pain relief after abdominal surgery, and significantly decreased the level of proinflammatory cytokines.

References:

1- Homburger JA, Meiler SE. Anesthesia, drugs, immunity, and long-term outcome. Curr Opin Anaesthesiology 2006; 19: 423 – 8

2- Watkins LR, Milligan ED, Maier SF – Glial proinflammatory cytokines mediate exaggerated pain states: implications for clinical pain. Adv Exp Med Biol, 2003; 521:1-21

3- Lin E, Lowr y SF. Inflammator y cytokines in major surger y: a functional perspective. Intensive Care Med 1999; 25: 255 – 7

4- Chachkhiani I, Gurlich R, Maruna P, Frasko R, Lindner J.   The postoperative stress response and its reflection in cytokine network and leptin plasma levels. Physiol Res 2005; 54: 279-85

5- Engelhardk, Werner C , and Eberspacher EThe effect of the α-2 agonist; dexmedetomidine and the NMDA antagonist; S (+) ketamine on the expression of apoptosis-regulating proteins after incomplete cerebral ischemia, reperfusion in rats. Aneth Analg 2003; 96: 524-31.

6- Snijdelaarh .B,Corneslisser ,Schmide C,and Katzl A randomized, controlled study of preoperative low dose S (+) ketamine in combination with postoperative patient controlled S (+) ketamine and morphine after radical prostatectomy. Anesthesia 2004; 98: 1385-1400.

7- KATZ J. Timing of preemptive analgesia, Clinical management of pain. London Arnold 2003; 113-62.

8- Meade P , Shoemaker W.C and Donelly i.T:Temporal patterns of hemodynamics, O_2 transport cytokines activity and complement activity in the development of adult respiratory distress syndrome after sever injury. J Trauma 1994; 36: 561-7.

9- Roytblat L, Talmor D, Rachinsky M, et al. Ketamine attenuates the interleukin-6 response after cardiopulmonary bypass. Anesth Analg 1998; 87: 266 –71.

10- Roytblat L, Roy-Shapira A, Greemberg L, et al. Preoperative low dose ketamine reduces serum interleukin-6 response after abdominal hysterectomy Pain Clin 1996; 9: 327–34.

11- Ilkjaer S, Nikolajsen L, Hansen TM, et al. Effect of i.v. ketamine in combination with epidural bupivacaine or epidural morphine on postoperative pain and wound tenderness after renal surgery. Br J Anaesth 1998; 81: 707–12.

12- Fu ES, Miguel R, Scharf JE. Preemptive ketamine decreases postoperative narcotic requirements in patients undergoing abdominal surgery. Anesth Analg 1997; 84: 1086 –90.

13- Tverskoy M,Oz verskoy M,Oz ,Isakson A,Finger J,Bradley EL.JR ,and Kisson I:Preemptive effect of fentanyl and ketamine on postoperative pain and wound hyperalgesia. Anesth Analg 1994; 78: 205-9.

14- Kawasaki C, Kawasaki T, Ogata M, Nandate K, Shigematsu A. Ketamine isomers suppress superantigen-induced proinflammatory cytokine production in human whole blood. Can J Anaesth 2001; 48: 819–23.

15- Hala Mostafa, Amr Mohamad Abo Ela and Nagwa El-Tweel. S (+) Ketamine Suppresses TNF-α, IL-6 and IL-8 Production in Blood in

Major Abdominal Surgery under Combined Epidural-General Anesthesia. *Journal of Medical Sciences* 2008; *8: 137-142.*